Riding Your Hormone Waves: How to Sync Your Lifestyle with Your Monthly Cycle

Riding Your Hormone Waves: How to Sync Your Lifestyle with Your Monthly Cycle

Copyright © 2024 by **Omolola Habib (NMD)**

Table of Content

Introduction

Have you ever felt like your body and mind are out of sync? One week you're riding high, getting everything done on your to-do list, and feeling great. But the next week, you're forgetful, overwhelmed, and can barely drag yourself out of bed.

Our hormones ebb and flow in cycles throughout each month. This is especially true for those who menstruate. The hormonal fluctuations of your menstrual cycle can significantly impact your mood, energy, productivity, and overall wellbeing if you don't know how to ride the waves.

This book will teach you how to leverage the natural rhythms of your body so you can unlock your potential, prevent burnout, and optimize your health every day of the month.

Cycle Syncing for Success

Women have a monthly cycle that follows the rise and fall of key reproductive hormones. Estrogen peaks mid-cycle, progesterone surges after ovulation, and both plummet during menstruation.

Most women just try to push through their cycle's ups and downs. They power through PMS, stress about missed periods, and chalk up their monthly symptoms as normal or "just hormones."

But your hormones are talking to you and sending you important messages! Each phase of your cycle has its own superpowers if you know how to work *with* your body's rhythms, rather than against them.

By syncing your lifestyle to your menstrual cycle, you can:

- Maximize energy, motivation, and productivity

- Lose weight and reduce PMS symptoms

- Enhance creativity and sense of wellbeing

- Deepen intimacy and relationships

- Prevent hormonal imbalances and burnout

Whether you're perimenopausal, menopausal, have irregular cycles, or are on birth control, you can benefit from cycle syncing. This book will help you tune into your body's wisdom so you can thrive through every phase.

What's Inside

In Part 1, we'll dive into the nitty gritty of your amazing menstrual cycle. I'll explain the role of each key hormone and teach you how to track your personal patterns and rhythms.

In Parts 2-5, you'll discover how to align your habits with each phase - follicular, ovulatory, luteal, and menstrual. You'll get phase-specific advice to maximize energy, productivity, fertility, and self-care.

Then in Parts 6-8, we'll cover how to sync your exercise, nutrition, and relationships to your cycle. I offer phase-specific workouts, meal plans, communication tips, and more to support your hormones.

By the end, you'll understand your body on a whole new level and have the tools to ride your hormone waves effortlessly.

A New Way of Living

I used to constantly fight against my body's natural rhythms, trying to keep up with unrealistic schedules and demands. I took the "push through your PMS" and "ignore your cramps" approach.

What I've learned is that when you work *with* your cycle, not against it, you free yourself from fighting your own body. Instead of struggling through each phase, you can flow through it with ease - a total game changer!

Are you ready to revolutionize your health and lifestyle by syncing with your natural cycles? Let's get started!

Chapter 1: Getting to Know Your Menstrual Cycle

Welcome to a whole new understanding of your amazing female body! In this chapter, we'll dig into everything you need to know about your menstrual cycle so you can start working with your natural rhythms.

Here's what we'll cover:

- The 4 phases of your cycle

- How estrogen, progesterone and other hormones fluctuate

- The role of your hypothalamus, pituitary gland, and ovaries

- How to track your unique cycle

- Common patterns and variations

- Busting myths and misconceptions

Let's start by looking at the basic anatomy of your menstrual cycle.

Menstrual Cycle 101

The menstrual cycle is the hormonal process of ovulation and menstruation that repeats every ~28 days for women of reproductive age.

Here are the main parts of your menstrual cycle:

- **Hypothalamus:** This is the control center in your brain. It releases GnRH (gonadotropin-releasing hormone).

- **Pituitary gland:** This communicates with your hypothalamus and ovaries. When prompted by GnRH, it releases FSH and LH.

- **Ovaries:** Your two ovaries take turns releasing an egg each cycle. They also produce key hormones like estrogen and progesterone.

- **Uterus:** Where a fertilized egg would implant and grow during pregnancy. Its lining builds up and sheds during your cycle.

Now, let's unpack how these parts work together in each phase of your cycle.

Phase 1: Follicular Phase

Length: ~14 days

The follicular phase starts on the first day of your period and ends when you ovulate. This phase is dominated by **estrogen**.

In the first part of the follicular phase, estrogen and FSH (follicle stimulating hormone) levels begin to rise. This triggers several ovarian follicles to start maturing. One becomes dominant and continues growing while the others die off.

As it grows, the dominant follicle produces more and more estrogen. This ramps up quickly in the last 1-2 days before ovulation.

During the follicular phase, you may notice:

- Light menstrual bleeding for 3-7 days

- Increasing cervical fluid and mucus

- Rising energy levels

- Heightened motivation and productivity

- Improved performance and endurance

- Enhanced creativity and sense of wellbeing

This is a great time to start new projects, exercise vigorously, socialize, and tap into your passion. We'll talk more about optimizing the follicular phase in Chapter 2.

Phase 2: Ovulation

Length: ~24-48 hours

When estrogen peaks, it triggers a surge of LH (luteinizing hormone). This causes the dominant follicle to burst and release its mature egg - ovulation!

Ovulation occurs around day 14 in a 28 day cycle, but can vary quite a bit. The egg then travels down the fallopian tubes toward the uterus.

Signs of ovulation may include:

- Sharp pain or cramps on one side of your pelvis/abdomen

- Increased libido

- Heightened senses, intuition and creativity

- Cervical fluid that's clear, slippery, and stretchy (like egg whites)

- Slight spotting

The 12-24 hours right before ovulation is when you're most fertile. We'll discuss how to identify your ovulation day and maximize this window in Chapter 3.

Phase 3: Luteal Phase

Length: ~14 days

After ovulation, the empty follicle turns into the corpus luteum and starts pumping out **progesterone**. Meanwhile, estrogen decreases but is still present.

Progesterone thickens the uterine lining and prepares it to receive a fertilized egg. If no implantation occurs, progesterone and estrogen plummet at the end of the luteal phase. This triggers menstruation and the start of a new cycle.

In the luteal phase, you may experience:

- Increased appetite and cravings

- More breast tenderness and bloating

- Sluggish digestion

- Fatigue and trouble concentrating

- Irritability and mood swings

- Clumsiness and brain fog

- Lower libido

For many women, PMS symptoms peak in the last days of the luteal phase. Self-care is key during this premenstrual week - more on this in Chapter 4.

Phase 4: Menstrual Phase

Length: ~3-7 days

With the corpus luteum gone, your hormone levels plunge. This causes your uterine lining to break down and shed - your period.

During menstruation you may notice:

- Heavy bleeding for a day or two, then lighter flow

- Cramps, headaches, fatigue

- Relief of PMS symptoms

- Low energy but increased creativity

- Minimal sex drive

It used to be advised to rest and limit activity during your period. But new research shows staying active can reduce pain and energetic. We'll get into managing your period in Chapter 5.

Getting to Know YOUR Cycle

Now that you understand the basic four phases, it's time to tune into your own unique menstrual cycle.

Here are three ways to get acquainted with your personal rhythms:

Track your periods

Marking the start and end dates of each period for several months helps you identify your average cycle length. You can use a calendar, app, or printable tracker.

Watch out for variability between cycles - it's normal to have a longer or shorter cycle occasionally. Tracking helps you notice when a big shift may signal issues like pregnancy, stress, or hormonal imbalances.

Check your cervical fluid

Observing your mucus patterns provides insight into where you are in your cycle, especially as you approach ovulation.

Right after your period, discharge is minimal. It increases as estrogen rises, becoming wetter and more slippery. Around ovulation, you'll see transparent, egg-white consistency cervical fluid. This fertile fluid allows sperm to survive.

Discharge then dries up and thickens during the luteal phase under progesterone's influence.

Monitor basal body temperature

Your basal or resting temperature spikes .5-1°F after ovulation due to progesterone.

Taking your temperature first thing in the morning and charting the reading pinpoints your ovulation date. The sustained temp rise confirms that the luteal phase has begun.

You may not need to track BBT long-term, but it's helpful upfront in understanding your cycle.

Common Variations

Now that you know the typical pattern, here are some natural variations you may experience:

Irregular cycles

It's normal for cycle length to vary occasionally. Stress, diet changes, illness, and travel can make your cycle shorter or longer at times.

If irregular cycles become your norm or you miss 3+ periods consecutively, see your doctor to rule out underlying issues.

Short and long cycles

Cycles between 21-35 days are clinically normal. Within that, short cycles often have shorter phases and long cycles have extended phases.

For instance, women with 21 day cycles tend to ovulate around day 7 rather than day 14. Their luteal phase is only 7-9 days.

Women with 35 day cycles ovulate around day 21 and have 16+ day luteal phases.

Luteal phase deficiency

A short luteal phase under 10 days may cause issues with implantation and fertility. However, minor variations in luteal length are normal.

Anovulatory cycles

It's normal to have an anovulatory cycle every once in awhile where no ovulation occurs. This leads to low/no progesterone and breakthrough bleeding.

If you have multiple anovulatory cycles in a row, see your doctor to identify potential hormonal imbalances.

Perimenopause and cycle changes

As you near menopause in your 40s, cycle irregularities are common due to waning ovarian function. This includes longer, shorter, and anovulatory cycles.

Busting Myths About Your Cycle

Now it's time to debunk some major misconceptions about the menstrual cycle:

Myth: Your period marks a "clean slate" when your hormones start over from zero.

Fact: Hormone levels fluctuate constantly and build upon one another. Estrogen begins rising in the follicular phase while you're still bleeding. There's no hormonal reset button each cycle!

Myth: Ovulation always occurs on day 14.

Fact: The day you ovulate varies based on your unique cycle length. Ovulation before day 10 or after day 17 is still considered normal and healthy.

Myth: PMS is imaginary or "in your head."

Fact: PMS is a genuine hormonal response. While impacts vary between women, the luteal phase brings valid physical and emotional changes.

Myth: Menopause means a total loss of femininity.

Fact: Your identity isn't defined by fertility or periods. Menopause brings positive hormone changes that liberate you from menstrual cycle fluctuations.

Myth: Birth control pills are just like your normal cycle.

Fact: Hormonal contraceptives prevent your natural hormone fluctuations, leading to different effects. We'll discuss birth control more in Chapter 7.

Core Messages

The key points to remember are:

- Your menstrual cycle follows a pattern of follicular, ovulatory, luteal, and menstrual phases.

- Estrogen dominates the follicular phase while progesterone peaks after ovulation.

- You can track your cycles by monitoring period dates, cervical fluid, and basal body temperature.

- It's normal to have some variations in cycle length and phase duration.

- Many myths and misconceptions exist about the menstrual cycle, but it helps to learn the facts.

Armed with a foundational understanding of your amazing menstrual cycle, you're ready to start optimizing each phase. Let's dive into the follicular phase next!

Chapter 2: The Follicular Phase

The follicular phase is prime time to socialize, start new projects, and exercise vigorously. Let's look at how to make the most of the rising estrogen superpowers during this first phase of your cycle.

We'll cover:

- Follicular phase hormones

- Energy levels and productivity

- Exercise and fitness

- Libido and sex

- Creativity and socializing

- Diet and nutrition

- Supplements and remedies

- Daily checklists

Grab your calendar and get ready to maximize the follicular phase!

Follicular Phase Hormones

The follicular phase starts on day 1 of your cycle when you get your period. It spans from menstruation until ovulation.

During this phase, **estrogen** begins to rise as ovarian follicles develop and mature. Estrogen peaks right before ovulation occurs.

Follicle stimulating hormone (FSH) also increases during the follicular phase. FSH recruits the follicles and stimulates their growth until one follicle becomes dominant.

By understanding these hormonal events, you can align your habits over the next two weeks.

Energy Levels and Productivity

Many women feel like superwomen during the follicular phase. Take advantage of this motivated and energetic window of time.

Focus on important projects

Estrogen helps dopamine rise, enhancing motivation and drive. Start new projects, tackle your to-do list, and make headway on big goals before your period begins.

Channel the extra energy into priorities rather than getting distracted. Avoid overscheduling yourself to prevent fatigue later in your cycle.

Maximize cognitive function

Estrogen boosts verbal fluency, memory, focus, and learning during the follicular phase.

Schedule brain-intensive tasks like presentations, exams, and interviews this first half of your cycle. The estrogen gives your cognition a bump.

Boost productivity habits

Create routines to optimize your work and productivity during the follicular phase.

Try block scheduling deep work sessions first thing in the morning when your willpower is highest. Or dedicate the afternoons for creative sessions or pumping out emails.

Adjust your habits each cycle to make the most of your follicular phase productivity powers.

Exercise and Fitness

The first half of your cycle offers peak athletic performance. Here's how to time your workouts:

Do high intensity exercise

Your lung capacity, endurance, and heart function improve as estrogen rises.

Aim for HIIT, running, cycling, and heavy strength training during the follicular phase. Go hard knowing your body can handle the increased intensity.

Avoid overtraining

Monitor your energy to avoid burnout. As estrogen declines approaching ovulation, back off the longest or most strenuous workouts.

Schedule a rest day when needed so you don't tap yourself out before the luteal phase.

Strengthen your pelvic floor

High estrogen helps increase blood flow and muscle mass. Make sure to incorporate kegels into your routine.

Aim for 3 sets of 10-20 reps daily to target your pelvic floor. This prevents incontinence and prepares your body for childbirth if that's in your future.

Stretch after hard workouts

Boost flexibility early in your cycle when your joints and tissues are more lax.

Focus on areas like hips, hamstrings, and shoulders. Dynamic stretching post-workout can enhance muscle repair.

Libido and Sex

Many women experience heightened arousal and libido as estrogen rises leading up to ovulation.

Have sex often

Take advantage of increased vaginal lubrication and sensitivity in the follicular phase. Extended foreplay feels great when estrogen is high.

Aim for more frequent sex or masturbation during this first half of your cycle if you feel desire.

Use lube as needed

While estrogen boosts lubrication, don't hesitate to use store-bought lubricant as well. This prevents uncomfortable friction.

Water-based lubes are ideal for condoms, while silicone-based lubes provide longer-lasting slick moisture.

Focus on self-pleasure

Even without a partner, nurture intimacy with yourself through self-touch. Explore what feels good physically and energetically.

Release oxytocin and opioids through orgasm's pleasurable contractions. This boosts your mood too!

Prioritize sexual health and pleasure to maximize this amorous phase.

Creativity and Socializing

Rising estrogen also activates your social butterfly during the follicular phase. Take advantage of increased dopamine and oxytocin early in your cycle.

Tap into your inspiration

Estrogen boosts divergent thinking, making room for creative breakthroughs.

Carve out time for your hobbies, passion projects or artists dates. Follow inspiration wherever it leads.

Organize social events

You'll likely feel more outgoing and chatty through the follicular phase. Plan get-togethers with friends or set up playdates for your kids.

Say yes to party invites and get excited about dressing up and being social.

Join a team or club

Sign up for a recreational sports league, hiking group, or book club to meet like-minded people. Forming new connections fires up your dopamine.

Look to volunteering and causes you care about too. Helping others releases the love hormone oxytocin.

Feed your social soul in the first half of your cycle when it craves community.

Diet and Nutrition

Tailoring your diet to the follicular phase can help you feel your best. Here's how to eat:

Eat more carbs

Good carbs provide energy for exercise and cognition. Enjoy starchy veggies, beans, fruit, and whole grains.

Time carb-heavy meals before intense workouts to fuel performance. Just don't overdo portions.

Stay hydrated

Drink plenty of water and herbal teas as estrogen levels rise. Hydration prevents headaches, bloating, and cramps.

Aim for at least eight 8-oz glasses of fluids daily, more if you exercise. Always sip water between alcoholic beverages too.

Add magnesium

Magnesium relaxes muscles and blood vessels, counteracting potential focal phase cramping.

Eat magnesium-rich foods like leafy greens, nuts, avocado, and whole grains. Or take 250-400 mg supplement before bed.

Reduce inflammatory foods

Avoid trigger foods like refined carbs, fried foods, and excess red meat and dairy. These can promote inflammation and acne.

Stick to a clean, nutrient-dense, anti-inflammatory diet through the follicular phase.

Supplements and Remedies

Certain herbs and nutrients offer extra follicular phase support:

Take a B-complex

B-vitamins give you an energy boost. Look for a B-complex with at least 25 mg B6 which helps reduce breast and facial bloating.

Try dong quai

This medicinal herb increases blood flow to your uterus and regulates menstruation. It minimizes heavy bleeding too.

Use evening primrose oil

EPO helps balance estrogen and alleviate PMS symptoms that may linger from your last period. It also boosts fertility.

Sip raspberry leaf tea

Raspberry leaf tones your uterus and can decrease menstrual cramps. Enjoy a cup or two per day.

Follicular Phase Checklist

To recap, here are smart strategies for the follicular phase:

- Tackle big projects and goals

- Maximize focus, drive, and cognitive function

- Do HIIT, endurance, and heavy strength training

- Have sex frequently when libido is up

- Feed creativity and social urges

- Eat carbs for energy, stay hydrated

- Take magnesium and B vitamins

- Use dong quai, EPO, or raspberry leaf tea

Tune into your energy levels as you move through the follicular phase. Adjust your self-care and habits flexibly based on how you feel day-to-day while making the most of rising estrogen.

Next let's look at honoring your body during the ovulatory phase. Get ready to pinpoint ovulation for fertility and creative insight!

Chapter 3: The Ovulatory Phase

Ovulation is a pivotal turning point each cycle. Let's explore how to identify ovulation and make the most of the 24-48 hour window around your estrogen peak.

Here's what we'll cover:

- How to pinpoint ovulation

- Fertility and conception

- Libido and sexual pleasure

- Energy levels and self-care

- Boosting creativity

- Honoring intuition and emotions

- Nutrition and exercise tips

It's time to harness the power of your ovulatory phase!

Pinpointing Ovulation

Ovulation occurs when a mature ovarian follicle ruptures and releases an egg, usually around cycle day 14. But the exact ovulation day varies by woman and cycle.

Here are signs ovulation is approaching:

- Increase in libido

- Breast swelling or tenderness

- Abdominal bloating

- Heightened senses and energy

Then right around ovulation you may notice:

- Mittelschmerz pain in your lower abdomen

- Spotting

- Wet, egg-white like cervical mucus

- Positive OPK test

Tracking your basal body temperature is the only way to confirm ovulation occurred. When your BBT spikes 0.5-1°F for 3+ days, you ovulated 1-2 days before the sustained rise.

Combining BBT with cervical fluid checks and an ovulation predictor kit can help identify your ovulation pattern. Over time you'll learn to recognize your pre-ovulation and peak fertility cues.

Fertility and Conception

The few days leading up to ovulation and the 24 hours after mark your most fertile window. Here are tips for conception:

Have well-timed sex

Target sex on your three peak fertile days based on cervical fluid and OPKs. Ensure sperm are ready to meet the egg.

However, don't let scheduled baby-making sex strain your relationship. Maintain intimacy through the process.

Support healthy cervical fluid

Fluid that stretches an inch or more signals peak fertility. Stay hydrated and minimize inflammatory foods so your mucus supports sperm motility.

Orgasm after ejaculation

Climaxes may help draw up sperm through uterine contractions. Though conception is possible without orgasm too.

Stay horizontal after sex

Laying down for 10-30 minutes post-sex allows more sperm to reach your cervix and avoid backflow.

Consider legs up against the wall

Some experts recommend getting your pelvis higher than your head after sex when trying to conceive. Experiment with positions that allow gravity to do its work.

Be patient through the process. Most healthy couples conceive within 6 months of well-timed sex during ovulation. See your doctor if you don't conceive after a year of focused efforts.

Libido and Sexual Pleasure

Many women find their libido peaks around the few days before and during ovulation. Tap into the natural increase in desire and arousal.

Have sex daily or every-other-day

If you're trying to conceive or just wanting intimacy, the days leading up to ovulation are prime time for love-making.

Incorporate self-pleasure

Masturbation helps you tune into your pre-ovulation arousal cues. Plus solo orgasms have fertility benefits by moving fluids and contractions.

Use positions that hit the G-spot

Deeper penetration targets the vaginal front wall. Woman-on-top and rear-entry positions provide G-spot stimulation.

Make time for playful connection

Flirt, massage each other, try sensual toys, play music to set the mood, and have fun. This builds anticipation leading up to ovulation.

Energy Levels and Self-Care

Tracking ovulation takes effort, so be sure to balance it with plenty of self-care.

Get good sleep

Prioritize 7-9 hours of sleep per night in the days surrounding ovulation. Quality rest ensures your cycle stays on track.

Relax and decompress daily

Try breathwork, meditation, Epsom salt baths, or calming poses to manage ovulation anticipation stress.

Ask for support if needed

Don't be afraid to reach out to your partner, friends, or support groups. Trying to conceive can be an emotional experience.

Listen to your needs around ovulation and speak up if certain strategies don't feel right for your body.

Boosting Creativity

Estrogen peaks at ovulation, bringing a surge of creative energy.

Capture inspiration and ideas

Keep a notebook handy to write down creative thoughts and inspirations near ovulation. Your innovative thinking is heightened.

Move your body freely

Free-form dance, improv exercise, and creative movement allow your inner artist to emerge. See what your body wants to express.

Play and experiment

Make time for fun creative play by fingerpainting, playing music, photography, or trying new artsy projects. Follow your muse.

Connect with your sacred feminine

channel this powerful fertile energy into your art, allowing your feminine spirit to flow through.

Honoring Intuition and Emotions

Alongside creativity, ovulation can amplify your emotions and intuition.

Tune into messages from your Higher Self

Quiet meditation and journaling around ovulation provides clarity. Listen to your inner wisdom.

Feel your feelings

Don't judge yourself if you feel more sensitive or tearful. Channel the emotions into artistic expression if needed.

Speak your truth

Powerful ovulatory hormones help you stand confidently in your worth and voice. Don't suppress yourself.

Trust your intuition

That inner knowing and gut instinct is strong at ovulation. Follow your hunches about people, opportunities, and decisions.

Nutrition and Exercise

Tailor your self-care around ovulation:

Choose nourishing foods

Focus on healthy fats, protein, and greens to stabilize hormones and energy. Savory tastes are satisfying.

Stay hydrated

Dehydration can disrupt ovulation. Sip water consistently and add electrolytes if you feel depleted.

Do lighter workouts

Avoid overheating and tapping yourself out. Walking, and swimming are great ovulatory exercise.

Apply warmth

Place a heating pad on your abdomen or lower back to ease any ovulation discomfort.

Hopefully these tips will help you pinpoint ovulation and fully embrace the magic of your ovulatory superpowers. Trust the wisdom of your body!

Next let's look at navigating the rollercoaster hormone changes of the luteal phase.

Chapter 4: The Luteal Phase

The luteal phase brings unique hormonal fluctuations that impact your mood, energy, and health habits. Let's look at thriving through this premenstrual part of your cycle.

We'll cover:

- Hormone changes

- Common PMS symptoms

- Coping with fatigue

- Managing mood swings

- Nurturing your body through discomfort

- Foods that help balance hormones

- Supplements to alleviate PMS

- Exercise dos and don'ts

- Week-by-week action steps

- When to see your doctor

This chapter will equip you with tons of tools to minimize the challenges of your luteal phase.

Luteal Phase Hormone Changes

The luteal phase starts right after ovulation and ends when your period begins, spanning cycle days 15-28.

The corpus luteum formed from your leftover follicle starts pumping out **progesterone** to thicken the uterine lining.

Estrogen declines after ovulation but is still moderately high during the first half of the luteal phase.

Together, elevated progesterone plus dropping estrogen trigger many premenstrual difficulties. But you can learn to ride these hormone waves skillfully.

Common PMS Symptoms

Up to 80% of menstruating women experience at least mild PMS discomforts as hormones fluctuate premenstrually.

Here are some of the most common luteal phase woes:

Physical symptoms: breast tenderness, bloating, headaches, cramps, acne, food cravings, fatigue

Mental/emotional symptoms: irritability, moodiness, anxiety, depression, trouble focusing, fuzzy thinking

Digestive symptoms: constipation, nausea, diarrhea, gas pain, indigestion

PMS severity varies widely between women based on hormone sensitivities and lifestyle factors. They often peak in the week before your period.

Learning your typical symptoms timeline helps you anticipate and mitigate them.

Coping With Fatigue

Extreme tiredness and low energy frequently arise during the luteal phase. Here are some tips:

Rest more

Nap daily if you can. Or at least put up your feet up to restore whenever possible. Leisurely walks can energize without tapping your reserves.

Go to bed earlier

Don't fight your growing need for sleep as progesterone rises. Gradually adjust your bedtime earlier, even by just 20-30 minutes.

Ask for support

Communicate your energy needs so your partner, family and coworkers understand if you need to offload tasks or work slower certain weeks.

Prioritize essentials

Scale back noncritical commitments to direct your limited energy toward priorities like work, childcare, and self-care.

Be compassionate with yourself. Extra rest recharges you to begin the follicular phase strong.

Managing Mood Swings

For many women, mood becomes a rollercoaster approaching their period due to shifting estrogen and progesterone.

Irritability, sensitivity, anger, sadness, and anxiety often spike, while joy, patience, and calm feel harder to access. A few coping strategies:

Catch mood shifts early

Learn your typical PMS mood patterns. At the first sign of irrational irritation or overreaction, regroup with self-care.

Avoid triggers

Minimize conflicts by laying low in situations that provoke your PMS reactions, like crowded spaces. Give yourself plenty of buffer room.

Talk it out

Voice your feelings to a trusted friend or therapist. Getting emotions off your chest prevents them from building up explosively.

Practice calming rituals

Make a list of things that soothe your nervous system, like aromatherapy, warm baths, nature walks. Use them preventively.

Forgive yourself

Don't beat yourself up over mood swings. Remind yourself it's just a phase, not a personality flaw.

Nurturing Physical Discomfort

From tender breasts to achy cramps, here are some ways to ease common luteal aches:

Use hot compresses

For breast tenderness or cramps, take a hot water bottle or heating pad to the area for pain-relieving warmth.

Try OTC pain relievers

Ibuprofen or acetaminophen can help minimize cramps and headaches as needed leading up to your period.

Massage tender zones

Ask your partner to rub your lower abdomen and back gently. Or use a tennis ball against tight muscles.

Soak in epsom salts

Magnesium-rich baths help relax pelvic tension and muscle spasms that contribute to cramping.

Go comfy

Wear loose clothing and skip constrictive bras and underwear that can aggravate pain zones.

Tune into your symptoms each cycle to find what comfort measures work best for you.

Luteal Phase Food Strategies

Diet tweaks can help balance your luteal phase hormones, energize, and curb cravings.

Increase protein

Eat protein with each meal, like fish, eggs, legumes, quinoa and nut butters. This stabilizes blood sugar and energy.

Choose complex carbs

Go for whole grains like oats, brown rice and buckwheat over processed carbs to minimize blood sugar spikes.

Load up on produce

Aim for 8-10 servings of antioxidant and fiber-rich fruits and veggies daily to decrease bloating.

Avoid salty foods

Minimize sodium for less fluid retention and swelling. Check labels for hidden salt.

Increase magnesium

Get more magnesium through spinach, nuts, avocado and beans or a 300-400 mg supplement. This eases muscle tension.

Stay hydrated

Drink plenty of fluid to counteract progesterone's dehydrating effect. Herbal tea offers hydration with soothing ritual.

Helpful Luteal Supplements

Certain herbs and nutrients are particularly beneficial for balancing hormones and easing PMS:

Evening primrose oil

EPO supplements provide essential fatty acids that promote hormone equilibrium. It takes about three months of consistent use to see effects.

Chasteberry

This herb reduces breast tenderness, bloating, irritability and other symptoms by supporting progesterone and estrogen balance.

Calcium and vitamin D3

These nutrients work synergistically to minimize pain, anxiety, and mood swings related to PMS. Take them together.

B6 or B-complex

B6 or a comprehensive B vitamin complex can relieve breast tenderness, fatigue, depression, nausea and headaches during PMS.

Discuss adding any new supplement with your healthcare provider, especially if you're on medication or trying to conceive.

Luteal Phase Exercise Dos and Don'ts

Your workouts require adjustment to match your energy and needs premenstrually.

DO: Low intensity movement

Gentle walks, leisurely cycling, pilates and swimming are ideal when your body is fatigued.

DO: Add stretching

Moves that open tight hips, chest and shoulders counteract PMS tension.

DO: Listen to your body

Cut back on exercise as needed based on how you're feeling. Be okay with taking more rest days.

DON'T: Push to exhaustion

Avoid HIIT workouts or heavy weights that wipe you out. Check your ego.

DON'T: Beat yourself up

Have compassion if your athletic performance declines before your period. Expect fluctuations.

DON'T: Work through pain

Skip exercise than aggravates breast tenderness or makes cramps worse.

Adjusting exercise prevents injury while still giving you mood-lifting movement.

Week-By-Week Action Steps

Now let's break down practical steps for self-care during the luteal phase:

Week 3 (Period Week)

- Continue eating clean and hydrating well

- Do gentle workouts like walking

- Rest and nap when needed; journal or vent feelings

- Take PMS supplements like magnesium and EPO

Week 4

- Gradually decrease workout intensity

- Add evening wind-down routines

- Eat more protein and healthy fats

- Take chasteberry or vitex if PMS gets severe

Week 1 (Premenstrual Week)

- Further reduce exercise; walk daily if possible

- Scale back nonessential tasks and events

- Connect with supportive friends; ask for help

- Apply heat; get massages for breast/pelvic discomfort

- Use OTC pain relievers as needed leading up to period

Tuning into your personal weekly patterns allows you to anticipate and treat symptoms proactively.

When to See Your Doctor

While most PMS discomfort is normal, contact your healthcare provider if:

- Symptoms severely disrupt work, relationships, or daily function

- Mood issues like depression persist throughout the luteal phase

- Cramping worsens and becomes intolerable

- Breast pain doesn't resolve with typical comfort measures

- You experience sudden cried spells or anxiety attacks

There are further medical options to explore if lifestyle remedies don't manage PMS adequately, such as medication or reproductive hormone testing.

I hope these tips equip you to care for your body with compassion as it moves through the luteal phase's ups and downs. You've got this!

It's nearly time for the monthly reset of your period. Let's talk optimal menstrual phase self-care next.

Chapter 5: The Menstrual Phase

The menstrual phase marks the turning of each cycle as your body sheds the uterine lining. Let's explore honoring your period for health, empowerment, and renewal.

We'll cover:

- Menstrual phase hormone changes

- Managing common symptoms

- Exercise tips

- Nutrition strategies

- Holistic remedies

- Hygiene and products

- Energy levels and self-care

- Creative outlets

- Rituals and spiritual practices

It's time to maximize the magic and meaning of your monthly bleed!

Menstrual Phase Hormone Changes

The menstrual phase spans the first 3-7 days of your cycle starting when you get your period. It continues until estrogen begins rising and new follicle growth resumes.

Your hormones are at rock bottom when your period begins:

- Estrogen and progesterone drop very low

- Follicle stimulating hormone (FSH) starts to increase

- Ovulation suppressing hormones like prolactin rise

This withdrawal triggers the shedding of your uterine lining as bleeding. These hormones fluctuations also cause common period symptoms.

Managing Menstrual Symptoms

For most women, menstrual symptoms peak in the first 1-2 days of their periods. Here are some remedies:

For cramps:

- Heat packs on your abdomen

- Over-the-counter pain relievers

- Orgasm and masturbation

- Calcium and magnesium supplements

- Anti-inflammatory foods

For heavy bleeding:

- Rest during flood days

- Take iron supplements if needed

- Drink plenty of fluids

- Add vitamin C foods to help absorption

For fatigue:

- Nap when possible

- Reduce commitments/expectations

- Move gently to energize

For headaches:

- Limit caffeine

- Try feverfew, ginger tea or peppermint essential oil

- Massage temples, neck and shoulders

Tune into your typical menstrual symptoms profile so you can customize relief each month.

Menstrual Exercise Tips

Moderate movement can help relieve menstrual woes. Here's how to modify workouts:

Keep exercising

Light to moderate activity, like walking and leisurely cycling, often reduces cramps and pain.

Avoid overexerting

During heavier flow days, take it easier with short, gentle workouts. Check in after exercise to ensure you don't feel wiped out or aggravated.

Slow down and stretch

Slower practices like Pilates target strength while preventing strain.

Pick comforting activities

If your usual exercise sounds unappealing premenstrually, opt for something grounding like easy hiking, swimming, or dance.

Listen to your body

Skip workouts that worsen pain or fatigue. Rest if needed.

Movement releases feel-good endorphins while preventing sluggishness. Find what works for your period.

Menstrual Nutrition Strategies

Tailor your diet to help minimize period symptoms:

Increase iron-rich foods

Beef, spinach, lentils, pumpkin seeds and quinoa supply iron to replace blood loss. Pair with vitamin C for absorption.

Reduce inflammation

Avoid trigger foods like refined carbs, excess sugar, and alcohol that can worsen pain and bloating.

Stay hydrated

Drink plenty of fluids and herbal teas to counter heavy bleeding dehydration.

Sip ginger tea

Ginger alleviates nausea, cramps, and migraines for many women.

Get more magnesium and calcium

These minerals relax muscles, calm nerves and reduce breast and uterine pain.

Indulge a little

Enjoy small treats if cravings strike. Just focus on nutrition overall.

Pay attention to how certain foods impact your unique period symptoms.

Holistic Remedies to Try

Herbs, essential oils, and other remedies can provide menstrual relief:

Cramp-easing supplements

Magnesium, calcium, and anti-inflammatory herbs like turmeric help relax the uterus.

Heat therapy

Try a rice sock heated in the microwave, hot water bottle, heating pad, or soak in a warm bath.

Essential oils

Rub diluted clary sage, rose, or lavender oil on your abdomen for pain and stress relief.

Orgasm

Climaxing releases tension in the pelvic area while contractions may expel blood faster.

Acupressure

Massaging the inner ankles, sacrum, or temples balances hormones and chi flow.

Experiment to find which holistic therapies provide you the greatest symptom alleviation.

Caring for Your Flow

Here are some tips for hygiene, comfort, and choosing period products:

Use the right pad or tampon absorbency

Change products every 4-6 hours, or more frequently on heavy days, for sanitation.

Consider a menstrual cup

Cups collect rather than absorb blood, creating less exposure to oxygen and chemicals.

Choose breathable cotton underwear

Avoid synthetics that trap heat and moisture against your vulva during your period.

Keep extras on hand

Carry an extra pad or tampon when out so you're prepared for surprises.

Shower regularly

Clean your vulva with mild soap and water at least daily. Avoid strong scented products.

Discard responsibly

Wrap used products securely before trashing them. Most offer discreet packaging.

Prioritize comfort and hygiene during your bleed. Don't hesitate to experiment with new period products to find your favorites.

Energy Levels and Self-Care

Be gentle with yourself on period days:

Rest when needed

Honor increased fatigue by napping, sleeping in, or going to bed earlier. Say no to extra obligations if possible.

Ask for help

Communicate your needs so your partner, family, and coworkers understand your energy fluctuations and pitch in more.

Reduce stressors

Minimize nonessential tasks and avoid stressful situations that can exacerbate PMS-like symptoms around your period.

Take time-outs

Step away to regroup when you feel overwhelmed. Even a few deep breaths in your car or a short walk around the block can provide relief.

Treat yourself to some extra pampering as your body works hard to shed your uterine lining.

Creative Outlets for Your Period

The surge of emotions and sensations on your period make it the perfect time to channel your inner artist. Here are some ideas:

Start a reflective journal

Writing about your journey, feelings, dreams, and needs is powerfully cathartic.

Craft or make art

Let your hands craft beauty from the intense emotions welling within. Paint, sculpt, knit, collage, or scrapbook.

Dance it out

Crank up music and move your body in free-form dance to get your energy flowing.

Take moody photos

Channel your dark and light sides into evocative photography. Play with shadows and light.

Make playlists

Curate menstrual music that captures your full range of complex moods and emptions.

Exploring creative mediums gives your inner world a voice during this potent time.

Rituals and Spiritual Practices

For thousands of years, societies celebrated feminine rites of passage around menarche and the moon cycle. Call on this lineage through ritual.

Create ceremonies

Design a monthly practice that affirms your womanhood. Include symbols of renewal that speak to you like flowers, fire, crystals, poetry, or mantra.

Tap into earth healing

Spend time in nature drawing on its grounding and replenishing energies as your body sheds what it no longer needs.

Meditate

Quiet contemplation helps calm emotions and reconnect with your inner wisdom during this transition.

Keep a goddess journal

Write letters to your future and past self. Jot down themes and lessons learned each cycle.

Craft moon altars

Decorate a sacred space using lunar imagery, goddess beads and charms, candles, stones, feathers, shells, crystals and more. Sit with it daily.

Ritual helps us find meaning in the mysterious, innate cycles of our bodies.

I hope these tips help you understand and care for your amazing menstrual phase. By working with your body's wisdom at this special time, you enable greater wellness all month long.

Onward now to exploring how diet powerfully interplays with your cycle...

Chapter 6: Food and Your Cycle

The right nutrition strategies can help you feel your absolute best at every phase of your cycle. Let's explore how to eat to stabilize hormones, boost energy, and alleviate symptoms.

We'll cover:

- General diet tips for cycle regulation
- Phase-specific meal plans
- Macronutrient recommendations
- Optimizing specific vitamins and minerals
- Foods to reduce PMS
- Managing cravings
- Recipes for each phase
- Supplements to support hormones
- When to see a dietitian

Follow along with the meal plans and prep some recipes to see just how powerful food can be in syncing your lifestyle to your natural rhythms.

General Diet Tips for Hormone Regulation

Certain nutrition principles help balance your hormones all month long:

Go for complex carbs

Choose whole grains like quinoa, brown rice, oats, and buckwheat instead of simple, processed carbs. Steady carbs prevent spikes and dips in blood sugar.

Increase plant protein

Incorporate legumes, nuts, seeds, and soy products to obtain protein with fiber for satiety. These support hormone pathways.

Load up on produce

Eat a rainbow of veggies and fruits to obtain a variety of vitamins, minerals and antioxidants that facilitate hormone function.

Healthy fats are essential

Obtain omega-3s from salmon, avocados, olive oil, chia seeds and walnuts for optimal hormone production.

Stay hydrated

Drink plenty of water throughout your cycle to avoid dehydration that can disrupt hormone balance. Herbal teas also hydrate.

Minimize added sugars

Keep desserts and sweets to occasional treats. Too much sugar leads to inflammation and estrogen dominance.

Reduce alcohol

Drink in moderation, especially in the luteal phase. Alcohol stresses the liver which metabolizes hormones.

Let's take a deeper look at tailoring your macros, vitamins, minerals and foods to find balance each phase.

Phase-Specific Macronutrient Needs

The optimum ratios of carbs, protein and fat fluctuate through your cycle based on your hormonal needs.

Follicular

Higher carb intake supports the energetic follicular phase. Aim for 50% carbs, 20% protein and 30% fat. Time carbs around workouts.

Ovulatory

Increase healthy fats like avocado and nuts to provide stability around ovulation. Try 40% carbs, 20% protein and 40% fat.

Luteal

Boost protein premenstrually, like fish, eggs and tofu, to prevent energy crashes. Aim for 40% carbs, 30% protein and 30% fat.

Menstrual

The ideal balance during your period is 45% carbs, 25% protein and 30% fat. Ensure sufficient iron-rich foods.

Listen to your body and fine-tune your personal macro ratios. Meal plans later in the chapter offer phase-specific guidance.

Optimizing Vitamins and Minerals

Certain micronutrients play key roles in menstrual cycle regulation. Be sure to obtain:

Vitamin B6

B6 helps balance estrogen and progesterone. Find it in poultry, potatoes, bananas, spinach, and hazelnuts.

Vitamin E

This antioxidant promotes estrogen balance. Eat seeds, nuts, spinach, and avocados to get your vitamin E.

Magnesium

Magnesium helps build progesterone and metabolize estrogen. Load up on leafy greens, nuts, and beans.

Calcium

Estrogen and calcium work synergistically. Include dairy, sardines, collard greens, fortified plant milks, and tofu.

Vitamin D

Low vitamin D is linked to estrogen dominance. Get your sunshine vitamin from eggs, fortified dairy, and mushrooms.

Iron

Iron supports ovulation and limits heavy periods. Meat, pumpkin seeds, lentils, and raisins can help avoid deficiencies.

Read labels and fill your diet with whole foods that offer bioavailable vitamins and minerals. Supplement selectively only after ensuring your diet is rich in these nutrients.

PMS-Busting Foods and Nutrients

Certain foods specifically help counteract premenstrual symptoms:

Salmon

The omega-3s in salmon improve mood, energy and skin health when estrogen dips premenstrually.

Chia and flaxseeds

Essential fatty acids from these seeds balance hormones and reduce breast tenderness and bloating.

Broccoli and cabbage

Cruciferous veggies contain compounds that help metabolize excess estrogen to treat PMS.

Bananas

Bananas are rich in potassium to reduce fluids retention as well as B6 for mood and cramps.

Yogurt with live cultures

The probiotics in yogurt support gut health for less PMS constipation and diarrhea. Choose plain, unsweetened varieties.

Be sure to incorporate these simple PMS fighters into your diet!

Strategies for Cravings

Intense food cravings commonly arise during the luteal phase as your hormones shift. A few smart ways to manage them include:

Indulge in moderation

Allow yourself small servings of the foods you crave without overdoing portions. This prevents rebound binging later.

Find healthier swaps

Substitute trail mix for chocolate, frozen yogurt for ice cream, fruit pops for candy. These provide satisfaction with more nutrition.

Stay hydrated

Thirst signals can disguise as hunger or cravings premenstrually. Drink plenty of water and herbal tea to stay satisfied.

Avoid trigger foods

Skip the vending machine if salty chips lead you down a vicious craving cycle. Control your environment.

Distract yourself

Go for a walk, call a friend, or immerse in a hobby when cravings hit to ride out the intensity peak.

Balancing your blood sugar throughout the day prevents crashes that exacerbate cravings. Time carbs, protein and fat wisely.

Sample Meal Plans for Each Phase

Now let's pull all these strategies together into sample meal plans tailored for each phase of your cycle!

Follicular Sample Meal Plan

Breakfast: Veggie egg white omelet with avocado toast

Snack: Greek yogurt with fruit and nuts

Lunch: Burrito bowl with brown rice, black beans, salsa, and guacamole

Snack: Energy bite made with oats, peanut butter, chocolate chips

Dinner: Grilled chicken, roasted sweet potato, and salad

Dessert: Berries with whipped cream

Ovulatory Sample Meal Plan

Breakfast: Smoked salmon, veggie and goat cheese omelet

Snack: Sliced apple with almond butter

Lunch: Lentil and kale soup with whole grain bread

Snack: Chia pudding made with coconut milk

Dinner: Veggie and tofu stir fry with cauliflower rice

Dessert: Dark chocolate avocado mousse

Luteal Sample Meal Plan

Breakfast: Kale and mushroom egg cups

Snack: Greek yogurt with pumpkin seeds and cinnamon

Lunch: Chicken, arugula and quinoa salad

Snack: Banana protein smoothie

Dinner: Turkey chili with butternut squash over baked potato

Dessert: Fresh berries

Menstrual Sample Meal Plan

Breakfast: Overnight oats with chia seeds, flax and fruit

Snack: Hardboiled egg and sauerkraut

Lunch: Lentil and brown rice soup with spinach salad

Snack: Carrots and hummus

Dinner: Grilled salmon, roasted Brussels sprouts and sweet potato

Dessert: Dark chocolate square

Tune in to your personal cravings and energy needs and modify these plans accordingly!

Recipes to Support Your Cycle

Eating seasonally and intuitively each phase will help you feel your best. To inspire you, here are nourishing recipes for each part of your cycle:

Follicular Recipes

[Follicular Recipes Here]

Ovulatory Recipes

[Ovulatory Recipes Here]

Luteal Recipes

[Luteal Recipes Here]

Menstrual Recipes

[Menstrual Recipes Here]

Hopefully these give you plenty of ideas to start cooking foods that align with your body's needs!

Supplements to Balance Hormones

In addition to a healthy diet, certain supplements provide extra support:

Follicular: B6, magnesium, omega-3s

Ovulatory: Vitamin C, omega-3s, magnesium

Luteal: B6, magnesium, calcium, Omega-3s, evening primrose oil

Menstrual: Iron, B12, folic acid, magnesium, omega-3s

Only supplement to fill in nutrient gaps not provided sufficiently through your whole food diet. Avoid megadoses.

Discuss supplement needs with your doctor, especially if pregnant or trying to conceive.

When to See a Dietitian

Meet with a registered dietitian if:

- You often feel weak, fatigued or dizzy

- Intense food cravings or hunger interfere with your life

- You suspect food sensitivities worsen symptoms

- Significant gastrointestinal distress accompanies your period

- Heavy bleeding contributes to iron deficiencies

- Fertility challenges may relate to diet issues

A nutrition expert can help personalize meal plans, recommend supplements, and identify potential dietary triggers related to your cycle. Invest in this support if needed!

Optimizing your diet provides one of the most powerful ways to sync your lifestyle to your female rhythms. Use this chapter as your guide to nourish yourself every phase.

Now let's explore how to align your exercise routine with your menstrual cycle...

Follicular Recipes

Energizing Oatmeal

- 1/2 cup rolled oats

- 1 cup milk of choice

- 1 tablespoon chia seeds

- 1 tablespoon almond butter

- 1/4 cup blueberries

- 1/4 teaspoon cinnamon

Cook oats in milk. Top with chia seeds, almond butter, blueberries and cinnamon.

Veggie Scramble

- 1 tablespoon olive oil

- 3 eggs, beaten

- 1/2 cup spinach

- 1/2 cup cherry tomatoes, halved

- 2 tablespoons feta cheese

- Salt and pepper to taste

Heat oil in pan. Add eggs and scramble until set. Fold in spinach and tomatoes. Top with feta. Season with salt and pepper.

Banana Protein Smoothie

- 1 banana, frozen

- 1 cup milk of choice

- 2 tablespoons peanut butter

- 1 scoop protein powder

- 1 tablespoon ground flaxseed

- Ice cubes

Blend all ingredients until smooth and creamy. Add ice to reach desired consistency.

Turkey Avocado Wrap

- 1 whole wheat tortilla

- 3 ounces sliced turkey

- 1/4 avocado, sliced

- 1/4 cup alfalfa sprouts

- 2 tomato slices

- 1 tablespoon hummus

Spread hummus on tortilla. Layer turkey, avocado, sprouts and tomatoes. Roll up tortilla.

Tuna Salad Stuffed Tomato

- 1 (5 ounce) can tuna, drained

- 2 tablespoons mayonnaise

- 1 celery stalk, diced

- 1 tablespoon dill

- 1 large tomato, cored

- 2 cups mixed greens

Mix tuna, mayonnaise, celery and dill. Stuff mixture into cored tomato. Serve on greens.

Chicken Quinoa Salad

- 1 cup quinoa, cooked
- 2 cups cooked chickpeas
- 1 grilled chicken breast, sliced
- 1 cup cherry tomatoes, halved
- 1 cucumber, diced
- 2 tablespoons balsamic vinaigrette

Combine quinoa, chickpeas, chicken, tomatoes and cucumber. Toss with vinaigrette.

Green Protein Smoothie

- 1 banana
- 1 cup kale
- 1 cup nut milk
- 1 scoop protein powder
- 1 tablespoon almond butter
- 1 tablespoon ground flaxseed
- Ice cubes

Blend all ingredients until smooth. Add ice to reach desired consistency.

Loaded Baked Sweet Potato

- 1 large sweet potato

- 1/4 cup black beans

- 2 tablespoons salsa

- 1/4 cup corn

- 2 tablespoons Greek yogurt

- 2 tablespoons shredded cheese

- Cilantro

Bake sweet potato. Top with beans, salsa, corn, yogurt, cheese and cilantro.

Cobb Salad

- 6 cups mixed greens

- 2 hardboiled eggs, sliced

- 2 turkey bacon strips, cooked and crumbled

- 1/2 avocado, sliced

- 1/4 cup blue cheese crumbles

- 2 tablespoons balsamic vinaigrette

Toss greens, eggs, bacon, avocado and blue cheese with vinaigrette.

Berry Protein Smoothie

- 1 cup almond milk

- 1 scoop vanilla protein powder

- 1 cup mixed frozen berries

- 1 tablespoon almond butter

- 1 tablespoon chia seeds

- Ice cubes

Blend all ingredients until smooth. Add ice to reach desired consistency.

Ovulatory Recipes

Veggie Frittata

- 1 teaspoon olive oil

- 3 eggs, beaten

- 1/2 cup baby spinach

- 1/4 cup cherry tomatoes, quartered

- 2 tablespoons crumbled feta cheese

Heat oil in ovenproof skillet over medium heat. Pour in eggs. Cook gently until edges begin to set. Top with spinach, tomatoes and feta. Broil 3-5 minutes until frittata is set.

Smoky Red Pepper Dip

- 1 (12 oz) jar roasted red peppers, drained

- 1/4 cup tahini

- Juice of 1 lemon

- 2 garlic cloves

- 1 teaspoon smoked paprika

- Salt to taste

- Vegetable sticks, for dipping

Blend peppers, tahini, lemon juice, garlic and paprika until smooth. Season with salt. Serve with veggie sticks.

Mason Jar Chopped Salad

- 1/2 cup quinoa, cooked
- 1/2 cup chickpeas
- 1/2 cup cucumber, diced
- 1/2 cup cherry tomatoes, halved
- 1 ounce feta cheese, crumbled
- 2 tablespoons balsamic vinaigrette

Layer quinoa, chickpeas, cucumber, tomatoes, feta and dressing in a mason jar. Shake before eating to mix.

Avocado Toast

- 1 slice whole grain bread, toasted
- 1/2 avocado, mashed
- 1 egg, cooked over-easy
- Salt and pepper to taste

Top toasted bread with mashed avocado. Top with over-easy egg and season with salt and pepper.

Mediterranean Tuna Salad

- 1 (5 ounce) can tuna, drained
- 1/4 cup tomato, diced
- 1/4 cup cucumber, diced
- 1/4 cup chickpeas, rinsed
- 2 tablespoons Greek yogurt
- 1 tablespoon lemon juice

- 1 tablespoon olive oil

- Salt and pepper to taste

In a bowl, mix tuna, tomatoes, cucumber, chickpeas, yogurt, lemon juice and olive oil. Season with salt and pepper.

Sheet Pan Salmon and Veggies

- 1 pound salmon fillet

- 2 cups broccoli florets

- 1 cup cherry tomatoes

- 1 tablespoon olive oil

- 1 teaspoon garlic powder

- 1 teaspoon paprika

- Lemon wedges

Toss broccoli and tomatoes with oil, garlic powder and paprika. Roast at 400F 10 minutes. Add salmon and roast 10 more minutes until fish flakes easily. Squeeze lemon over top.

Chia Pudding

- 1/4 cup chia seeds

- 1 cup coconut milk

- 1 teaspoon vanilla

- 1 tablespoon honey or maple syrup

- 1/2 cup mixed berries

In a container, combine chia seeds, milk, vanilla and honey. Refrigerate overnight. Top with berries before serving.

Mediterranean Stuffed Peppers

- 4 bell peppers, tops removed
- 1 (15 ounce) can chickpeas, drained and rinsed
- 1 cup cooked quinoa
- 1/2 cup crumbled feta cheese
- 1/4 cup sliced kalamata olives
- 2 tablespoons lemon juice
- Salt and pepper to taste

Mix chickpeas, quinoa, feta, olives and lemon juice. Season with salt and pepper. Stuff mixture into pepper halves. Bake at 375F for 25 minutes.

Green Goddess Smoothie

- 1 cup spinach
- 1 cup coconut water
- 1/2 avocado
- 1/2 banana
- 1 tablespoon almond butter
- 1 tablespoon chia seeds
- 1 tablespoon honey
- Ice cubes

Blend all ingredients until smooth. Add ice to reach desired consistency.

Luteal Recipes

Tofu Scramble

- 1 tablespoon olive oil
- 1 block firm tofu, crumbled
- 1/2 bell pepper, diced
- 1/4 cup mushrooms, sliced
- 1/4 onion, diced
- 1/2 cup spinach
- 2 tablespoons nutritional yeast
- 1/2 teaspoon turmeric
- Salt and pepper to taste

Heat oil in pan over medium heat. Add tofu, bell pepper, mushrooms and onion. Cook 5 minutes until softened. Add spinach and cook 1 more minute. Stir in nutritional yeast and turmeric. Season with salt and pepper.

Protein Overnight Oats

- 1/2 cup rolled oats
- 1/2 cup milk of choice
- 1 tablespoon chia seeds
- 1 tablespoon peanut butter
- 1/2 scoop protein powder
- 1/4 cup blueberries

In a container, combine oats, milk, chia seeds, peanut butter, protein powder and blueberries. Refrigerate overnight.

Veggie Rice Bowl

- 1 cup cooked brown rice
- 1/2 cup black beans
- 1/2 cup roasted sweet potato
- 1/2 cup sautéed kale
- 2 tablespoons avocado
- Lime wedge

Assemble rice, beans, sweet potato, kale and avocado in a bowl. Squeeze lime juice over top.

Chicken Zoodle Soup

- 2 chicken breasts, cooked and shredded
- 2 large zucchinis, spiralized
- 4 cups chicken broth
- 1 (15 ounce) can diced tomatoes
- 2 celery stalks, chopped
- 1 tablespoon Italian seasoning
- Salt and pepper to taste

Simmer zoodles in broth 2 minutes. Add chicken, tomatoes, celery and seasoning. Cook until warmed through.

Lentil Salad

- 1 cup cooked lentils

- 1 cup chopped cucumber

- 1/2 cup halved cherry tomatoes

- 1/4 cup crumbled feta

- 2 tablespoons balsamic vinaigrette

- Salt and pepper to taste

Toss lentils, cucumber, tomatoes and feta with vinaigrette. Season with salt and pepper.

Sheet Pan Lemon Chicken

- 4 boneless skinless chicken breasts

- 1 pound brussels sprouts, halved

- 2 tablespoons olive oil

- 2 tablespoons lemon juice

- 1 teaspoon garlic powder

- 1 teaspoon dried oregano

- Salt and pepper to taste

Toss brussels sprouts with 1 tablespoon oil. Roast at 400F for 10 minutes. Toss chicken with remaining oil, lemon juice and seasonings. Add to pan and roast 15 minutes until chicken is cooked through.

Banana Oat Muffins

- 1 3/4 cups oats

- 2 bananas, mashed

- 2 eggs

- 1/3 cup milk

- 1/3 cup peanut butter

- 1 teaspoon baking soda

- 1 teaspoon cinnamon

- 1/2 cup mix-ins like nuts or chocolate chips

Blend oats into a flour. Mix bananas, eggs, milk, peanut butter, baking soda and cinnamon. Fold in oat flour and mix-ins. Scoop batter into a greased muffin tin. Bake at 350F for 18-20 minutes.

Mediterranean Baked Salmon

- 1 pound salmon fillet

- 1 tablespoon olive oil

- 2 garlic cloves, minced

- 1 teaspoon dried oregano

- 1/4 cup cherry tomatoes, halved

- 1 lemon, sliced

- Salt and pepper to taste

Place salmon in baking dish. Drizzle with oil and top with garlic, oregano, tomatoes and lemon slices. Season with salt and pepper. Bake at 400F for 12-15 minutes until cooked through.

Matcha Smoothie

- 1 banana

- 1 cup milk of choice

- 2 tablespoons almond butter

- 1 tablespoon matcha powder

- 1/2 cup ice

Blend all ingredients until smooth and creamy.

Chicken and Vegetable Soup

- 1 tablespoon olive oil
- 1 pound boneless skinless chicken breasts, diced
- 1 onion, diced
- 3 carrots, sliced
- 3 stalks celery, sliced
- 1 zucchini, sliced
- 6 cups chicken broth
- 2 bay leaves
- 1 cup rice or pasta
- Salt and pepper to taste

Heat oil in a pot. Cook chicken until no longer pink. Add onion, carrots, celery and zucchini. Cook 5 minutes. Add broth and bay leaves. Simmer 20 minutes. Remove bay leaves. Add rice or pasta and cook until tender, 10-15 minutes. Season with salt and pepper.

Menstrual Recipes

Scrambled Tofu

- 1 tablespoon olive oil
- 1 package firm tofu, crumbled
- 1/2 red bell pepper, diced
- 2 cups fresh spinach
- 2 tablespoons nutritional yeast

- 1/4 teaspoon each turmeric, cumin, paprika

- Salt and pepper to taste

Heat oil in pan over medium heat. Add tofu and cook 5 minutes. Add bell pepper and spinach and cook 2 minutes more. Stir in spices and cook 1 minute. Season with salt and pepper.

Avocado Toast

- 1 slice whole grain bread, toasted

- 1/2 mashed avocado

- 1/2 tablespoon everything bagel seasoning

- 1 egg, cooked over-easy

Mash avocado onto toasted bread. Sprinkle with bagel seasoning. Top with over-easy egg.

Roasted Root Vegetables

- 2 carrots, chopped

- 2 parsnips, chopped

- 1 sweet potato, chopped

- 1 red onion, chopped

- 2 tablespoons olive oil

- 1 teaspoon dried rosemary

- Salt and pepper to taste

Toss carrots, parsnips, sweet potato and onion with olive oil. Sprinkle rosemary and season with salt and pepper. Roast at 425F for 25-30 minutes, until tender.

Lentil Stew

- 1 tablespoon olive oil

- 1 onion, diced

- 3 carrots, sliced

- 3 celery stalks, sliced

- 1 cup dried lentils, rinsed

- 1 (14 ounce) can diced tomatoes

- 4 cups vegetable broth

- 2 bay leaves

- 1 teaspoon paprika

- 1 teaspoon cumin

- Salt and pepper to taste

In a pot, sauté onions, carrots and celery in oil 5 minutes. Add lentils, tomatoes, broth and spices. Simmer 30 minutes until lentils are tender. Discard bay leaves. Season with salt and pepper.

Sheet Pan Salmon

- 1 pound salmon fillet

- 2 cups Brussels sprouts, halved

- 2 cups butternut squash, chopped

- 2 tablespoons olive oil

- 1 teaspoon dried thyme

- Salt and pepper to taste

Toss Brussels sprouts and squash with oil. Season with thyme, salt and pepper. Roast at 400F for 10 minutes. Push veggies to edges, add salmon to center and roast 10-15 minutes more until cooked through.

Wild Rice Pilaf

- 1 cup wild rice

- 2 cups vegetable broth

- 1 onion, diced

- 2 carrots, diced

- 2 celery stalks, diced

- 1/2 cup toasted pecans

- 2 tablespoons fresh parsley, chopped

- Salt and pepper to taste

Bring rice and broth to a boil, then reduce to a simmer. Cook 45 minutes until rice is tender. Remove from heat and add vegetables and pecans. Season with salt and pepper. Let stand 5 minutes before serving.

Blueberry Cobbler

- 2 cups blueberries

- 1 tablespoon lemon juice + zest

- 1/3 cup sugar

- 1 cup flour

- 1/4 cup oats

- 6 tablespoons butter, divided

- 1 teaspoon baking powder

- 1/4 cup milk

- Cinnamon sugar

Toss blueberries with lemon juice and zest. Add sugar and let sit. Mix flour, oats, 4 tablespoons butter, baking powder, pinch of salt. Cut in remaining butter. Stir in milk. Drop dough over fruit. Top with cinnamon sugar. Bake at 375F for 25 minutes.

Veggie Chopped Salad

- 2 cups chopped romaine

- 1/2 cup canned chickpeas, rinsed

- 1/2 cup cherry tomatoes, halved

- 1/2 cucumber, sliced

- 1/4 cup grated carrot

- 1 ounce feta cheese, crumbled

- Balsamic vinaigrette

Toss together lettuce, chickpeas, tomatoes, cucumber, carrot and feta. Dress with desired amount of vinaigrette.

Carrot Ginger Soup

- 1 tablespoon olive oil

- 1 onion, chopped

- 3 large carrots, chopped

- 1 tablespoon fresh ginger, grated

- 3 cups vegetable broth

- Salt and pepper to taste

Heat oil over medium heat. Add onion and cook 5 minutes until softened. Add carrots and ginger and cook 2 minutes more. Pour in broth and simmer 20 minutes until carrots are very soft. Puree soup with blender or immersion blender. Season with salt and pepper.

Chapter 7: Exercise and Your Cycle

Physical activity is an essential piece of caring for your body across your menstrual cycle. Let's discuss how to modify your workouts to match your monthly needs and capacities.

We'll cover:

- Overall exercise benefits

- Customizing workouts each phase

- Matching intensity to energies

- Sample workouts for each phase

- signs to reduce activity

- addressing amenorrhea

- strategies for athletes

Follow along with the workouts that align with where you're at in your month!

Overall Exercise Benefits

Consistent exercise lengthens your cycle phases promoting hormonal balance. Additional benefits include:

- Increased ovulation regularity

- Reduced PMS and cramps

- Less pain and heavier bleeding during your period

- Improved mood and energy throughout your cycle

- Help coping with menopause transition symptoms

- Building bone density to prevent osteoporosis

Aim for at least 150 minutes of moderate exercise per week, along with strength training twice weekly. Move daily if possible!

Customizing Workouts for Each Phase

Tailoring workout intensity and types to your cycle maximizes gains while preventing overexertion.

Follicular

Focus on higher intensity during the energetic follicular phase when estrogen peaks.

Ovulatory

Lower intensity workouts around ovulation prevent stressing your reproductive system.

Luteal

Reduce duration and exertion during the luteal phase as energy dips and body feels more sensitive.

Menstrual

Gentle exercise relieves cramping during your period, but rest as needed.

Matching Intensity to Your Energy Levels

Tune into your energies and calibrate exertion accordingly:

High Energy Periods - Follicular and ovulatory phases

- Prioritize high intensity interval training

- Lift heavy weights and increase reps

- Sprint or run at maximum speeds

- Take advanced fitness classes

- Play recreational sports

- Challenge your capacities

Lower Energy Periods - Luteal and menstrual phases

- Focus on walking, swimming

- Choose beginner classes and lighter weights

- Keep workouts under an hour

- Do lower intensity cardio intervals

- Try restorative stretching or Pilates

- Listen and back off at the first signs of fatigue

Honor where your body is at each week without judgment. Adjust intensity fluidly across your cycle.

Sample Workouts for Each Phase

Here are a variety of workouts to try in each part of your cycle:

Follicular Sample Workouts

Strength: Complete a circuit going hard for 30 seconds at each station - planks, mountain climbers, push-ups, squat jumps, lateral lunges, burpees. Repeat for 4-5 rounds.

Cardio: Run 1 minute at your fastest sprint pace, 1 minute at marathon pace, repeat 5x. Or bike, rowing machine, or swim instead.

Cross-training: Take a high-energy aerobics class like Zumba. Do a bootcamp class with stations and weights. Play a competitive sport like volleyball or basketball.

Ovulatory Sample Workouts

Strength: Do 2-3 sets of 8-12 reps per move at a weight that allows full form. Try goblet squats, shoulder presses, bent-over rows, and split squats.

Cardio: Go for a 45 minute run, cycle, swim or elliptical session at a moderate, challenging pace you can sustain. Get outside!

Cross-training: Enjoy an aqua-fitness class at your own intensity level if you have access to a pool.

Luteal Sample Workouts

Strength: Try 2 lighter sets of 12-15 reps of moves like deadlifts, lateral raises, chest press and hip thrusts. Focus on correct form.

Cardio: Keep your heart rate under your typical max doing intervals - 2 min hard effort, 1 min recovery x 10 rounds. Or go on a hike outdoors.

Cross-training: Take a beginner Pilates video or class emphasizing core strength. Try barre exercises to increase lean muscle mass.

Menstrual Sample Workouts

Strength: Use lighter weights for 1-2 sets of 15-20 reps of glute bridges, front squats, bicep curls and tricep dips. Or take a rest day.

Cardio: Walk at an incline on the treadmill or outdoors if weather permits. Go for 30-40 minutes.

Cross-training: Take a leisurely swim, focusing on form. Do gentle cycling or the elliptical at moderate effort.

Try these workouts or modify them to fit your needs and interests each phase. Honoring your cycle doesn't mean rigidly sticking to a plan every month if it doesn't feel right. Stay responsive to your body's wisdom.

Listening to Your Body

Stay attuned for signals to pull back on exercise:

- Extreme fatigue or dizziness

- Shortness of breath

- Pelvic or abdominal pain

- Worsening PMS symptoms

- Irregular period onset or intensity

- Injury risk due to low coordination

Honor when your body asks for more rest. Pushing excessively can disrupt your hormones and cycle!

Addressing Amenorrhea

If you stop getting your period consistently, especially coupled with intense exercise training, you may have exercise-induced amenorrhea.

This reproductive system issue arises from energy deficits and stress hormones suppressing ovulation. Aim to correct it through:

- Increasing calorie intake, especially carbs

- Reducing excess cardio exercise

- Managing workout stress

- Adding recovery days

- Improving sleep quantity and quality

See your doctor for evaluation and supervision if menstrual irregularities persist despite lifestyle adjustments.

Tips for Athletes

Female athletes require tailored support across their cycle:

- Track your cycle religiously using clues like temperature and cervical fluid to ensure you're ovulating

- Meet with a sports dietitian to optimize your nutrition

- Structure intense training around the follicular and ovulatory phases when your body can handle it

- Listen to your luteal and menstrual needs to incorporate active recovery

- Meet with a coach or trainer who understands the female body

Take care not to overtrain or underfuel. Nurture synchronization with your natural rhythms to prevent injury and burnout.

I hope these tips help you leverage exercise for optimal energy and wellbeing all month long! Check in with what your body needs across your unique menstrual journey.

Chapter 8: Your Cycle and Relationships

Your menstrual cycle influences how you relate to others and vice versa. Let's explore navigating relationships across your changing monthly rhythms.

We'll cover:

- Impacts on communication

- Libido and intimacy fluctuations

- Changing moods and needs

- Strengthening partnerships

- Sex during your period

- Hot flashes and relationships

- Supporting daughters and mentees

- Fostering community and belonging

- Working with changing energies

Understanding your relational patterns across your menstrual journey can help you build deeper bonds with those you love.

Communication Shifts

The hormones of each phase shape your social capacities—for better or worse! Estrogen and oxytocin make the follicular phase prime socializing time, while premenstrual drops in serotonin can hinder positive communication.

Follicular communication style:

- Upbeat, chatty, outgoing

- Articulate and thoughtful

- Confident speaking up about needs

- Not as sensitive to criticism

Ovulatory communication style:

- Increased perception and intuition

- Desire for meaningful connection

- Ability to read nonverbal cues

- More emotional sensitivity

Luteal communication style:

- Increased irritability and reactions

- Difficulty finding words

- Heightened sensitivity to conflict

- More introverted and withdrawn

Menstrual communication style:

- Quieter and more reflective

- Difficulty concentrating on conversations

- Emotional sensitivity and tears

- Need more personal space

Share these patterns with loved ones so they understand your varying social capacities across the month.

Navigating Monthly Libido Shifts

Your interest in sensuality and sexual intimacy changes as hormones fluctuate.

Libido often spikes leading up to ovulation, when estrogen is high and cervical mucus facilitates reproduction.

However, everyone has a unique monthly rhythm. Work with your natural currents of desire, communicating your needs sensitively with your partner.

Use the lower libido times to focus on emotional intimacy - cuddling, giving massages, sharing vulnerably, planning romantic dates out, and expressing affection through words and gifts.

Prioritize sexual pleasure across the month in ways that feel good for you both physically and emotionally.

Coping with Changing Moods

Shifting progesterone and estrogen impacts mood dramatically for many women. Irritability and sensitivity peak for several days before your period begins.

Here are some tips for smoothing relationships with partners and family when PMS emotions run high:

- Give them the heads up your period is coming so they're forewarned

- Have an agreed upon word you can say when you need to disengage and cool down, like "pineapple" or "pepper."

- Carve out some alone time when you feel on the brink of losing your cool

- Ask them to go for a walk with you to get fresh air and move your body

- Request extra support with household obligations that feel overwhelming

- Plan relaxing activities leading up to your period like massages, baths and reading

- Verbalize when you notice your reactions feel irrational and apologize

- Use humor to diffuse tense moments when possible

While challenging, reminding yourself the moodiness will pass soon helps you ride the wave.

Strengthening Partnerships

All relationships benefit when each partner understands and supports the other's cycle. Try:

Educating them on the process: Explain your four phases and associated patterns. Share resources so they learn with you.

Communicating needs clearly: Don't expect them to be a mind-reader each month. But do speak up about energetic or emotional support needed.

Making requests early: Give advance notice before the luteal phase so they can be proactive - like planning date nights earlier in the month.

Showing appreciation: Express gratitude for their efforts and partnership during more challenging times of the month.

Doing self-work: Take personal responsibility through journaling, therapy, and self-care practices to prevent making them your punching bag.

Healthy relationships let each person feel seen and supported through life's inevitable ups and downs. Foster this mutuality around your cyclic journey.

Is Sex During Your Period Right for You?

Some couples enjoy the natural lubrication and the intimacy of period sex, while others wait until it has passed—both are perfectly normal!

If you want to give it a try, here are some tips:

- Place towels underneath to catch any blood
- Use a menstrual cup to minimize flow during sex
- Stick to positions that limit mess and discomfort
- Make it a gentle, slow experience
- Shower together afterwards
- Follow your instincts - stop if it doesn't feel right

Keep the lines of communication open about needs and comfort levels.

Navigating Hot Flashes with Loved Ones

The hormonal havoc of perimenopause and menopause brings on hot flashes - that sudden feeling of feverish heat accompanied by flushing and sweats.

Here's how to minimize their social disruption:

- Carry a portable handheld fan to cool off promptly
- Dress in breathable, removable layers
- Avoid common hot flash triggers like caffeine, alcohol, excess heat, and spicy foods
- Explain in advance it's just a temporary menopause symptom
- Crack jokes to ease any awkwardness
- Have a water bottle handy to rehydrate
- Be patient but enforce boundaries if comments turn insensitive

Regular exercise, stress management, and hormone balancing lifestyle habits can help reduce hot flash intensity over time as well. You've got this!

Supporting Daughters and Mentees

If a young girl or teen in your life starts menstruating, she needs compassion and practical guidance. Offer:

- An understanding ear without judgment or shaming
- Resources to learn about the menstrual cycle
- Tips for tracking her cycles, interpreting her symptoms, and caring for her body
- Reassurance discomforts and emotions are normal
- Help determining when a doctor visit might be needed
- The confidence to advocate for herself at school/work

Also:

- Make sure she has needed period supplies and pain remedies
- Remind her to exercise and eat a healthy diet
- Suggest ways to soothe PMS like hot pads, tea, baths
- Share your own experiences so she doesn't feel alone or defective

Model self-acceptance, body literacy, and care as she navigates periods.

Fostering Community and Belonging

Your menstrual experience can connect you with others. Consider:

Talking openly about periods: This normalizes a natural process and dismantles taboos. Share your ups and downs!

Attending gatherings focused on cycles: Goddess circles, women's circles, moon lodges, and retreats offer ritual and wisdom. Red Tents gather women to share their menstrual journeys.

Joining online groups: Connect through forums and social media with those on a similar path worldwide. Follow educators on women's health topics.

Volunteering with organizations: Look for nonprofits like I Support the Girls that supply period products to those in need and empower cycle understanding.

Practicing sisterhood self-care: Do spa nights, and cooking with girlfriends. Celebrate your place in the lineage of womanhood.

Lean on your sisters when your body needs extra love. Turn to communities aligning with your cyclical nature.

Working with Your Monthly Energy

Your professional and creative energies rise and fall across your menstrual cycle. Leverage your natural productivity rhythms:

Track when you feel most in flow – your ideas pour out effortlessly. Do your deepest work then.

Honor when your brain feels foggy – Be okay with just getting mundane tasks done during these times. Don't force creativity or complex problem solving.

Communicate needs transparently – Explain you have cyclical patterns that impact your working pace and style.

Take time off if possible – See if you can work from home or flex your schedule on heavy days. Even an afternoon nap can turn the tide.

Hold creativity loosely – Inspiration will return; be patient with fallow periods knowing you must rest to renew.

Work with instead of against your natural currents to prevent fatigue. Ride each cycle's productivity wave skillfully.

Hopefully these tips help you nurture relationships with understanding and compassion across your amazing menstrual journey. Share your truth gently but unapologetically.

Conclusion: Living in Sync with Your Cycles

We've covered a lot of territory together exploring how to sync your lifestyle to your menstrual cycle for greater energy, comfort, and empowerment.

By now you have a strong foundation in:

- The four menstrual phases and their hormonal patterns

- Optimizing each week of your cycle through nutrition, exercise, self-care practices, and relationships

- Tuning into your personal rhythms, symptoms, and shifts

- Working with your natural currents instead of against them

- Leveraging the superpowers and capacities of each phase

I hope this book has helped you become more body literate, appreciating your cycle as an asset rather than an inconvenience to manage.

While our hormone fluctuations as women are often framed negatively, they offer us unique gifts and insights when worked with skillfully.

Your menstrual cycle provides a portal to tune into your emotional, physical and spiritual needs each month. It invites you to rest and restore as well as push your edges when the timing is right.

You now have an abundance of tools and resources to deepen this relationship with your cyclical self.

Yet this journey requires practice, patience, and self-compassion. There will be off months when things feel chaotic or out of sync. Give yourself plenty of grace as you learn your unique rhythms.

Cycle syncing is a lifelong process of listening to your inner wisdom and loving your body through every up, down, and turn.

Each new phase of your menstrual life like pregnancy, postpartum, breastfeeding, and perimenopause requires relearning your body's cues all over again.

The core principles remain the same—care for yourself exquisitely through each rise and fall, tuning into the guidance of your hormones and energies.

Trust in your abilities to become fluently cyclic. Allow this process to blossom your mind-body connection and feminine empowerment.

You've got this! Here's to riding your natural hormone waves with ease, joy, flow, and vitality.

www.ingramcontent.com/pod-product-compliance
Lightning Source LLC
Chambersburg PA
CBHW061000260726
48661CB00005B/1971